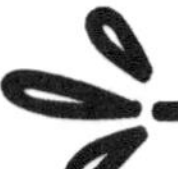

Thank you for purchasing our book.
We hope you love it!

"MAKING SMALL CHANGES TO YOUR DIET CAN MAKE A BIG DIFFERENCE"

This book belongs to

Copyrights©

This content is copyright of
Maples Book Solutions© 2024.
All rights reserved.

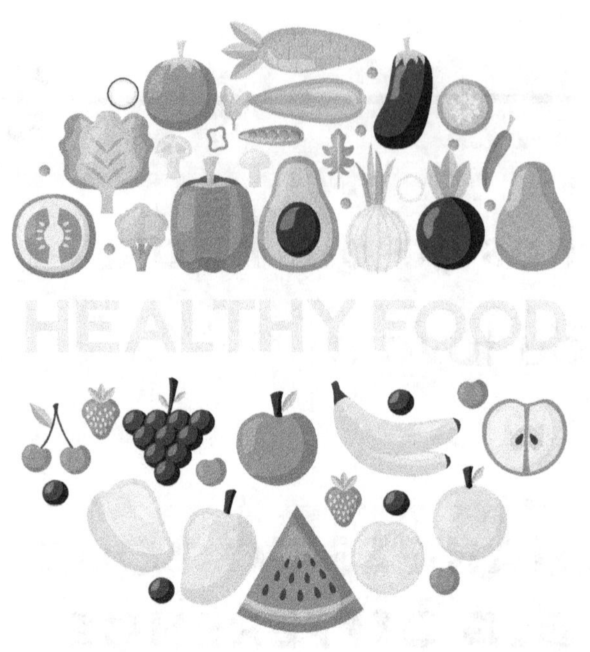

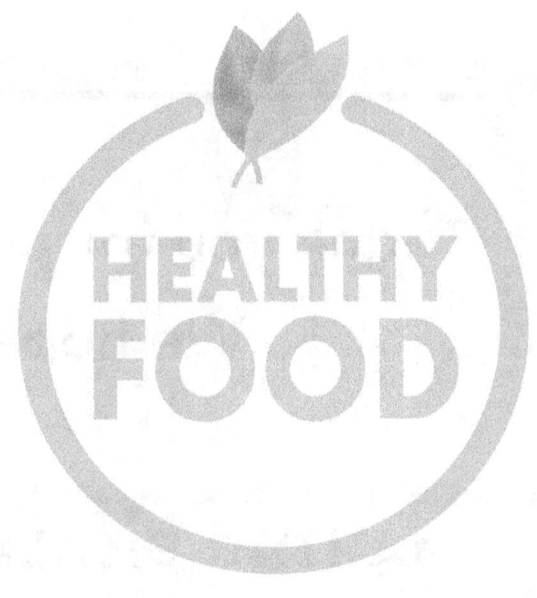

HOW TO EAT RIGHT TO BE HEALTHY AND ENERGETIC

TIPS AND TRICKS FOR ALL AGES

1. Diversify your diet.
2. Drink enough water.
3. Reduce sugar and salt intake.
4. Eat more protein
5. Reduce the amount of fat.
6. Eat foods rich in vitamins and minerals.
7. Do not forget about healthy sleep.

5 STEPS TO MAINTAIN
YOUR HEALTH

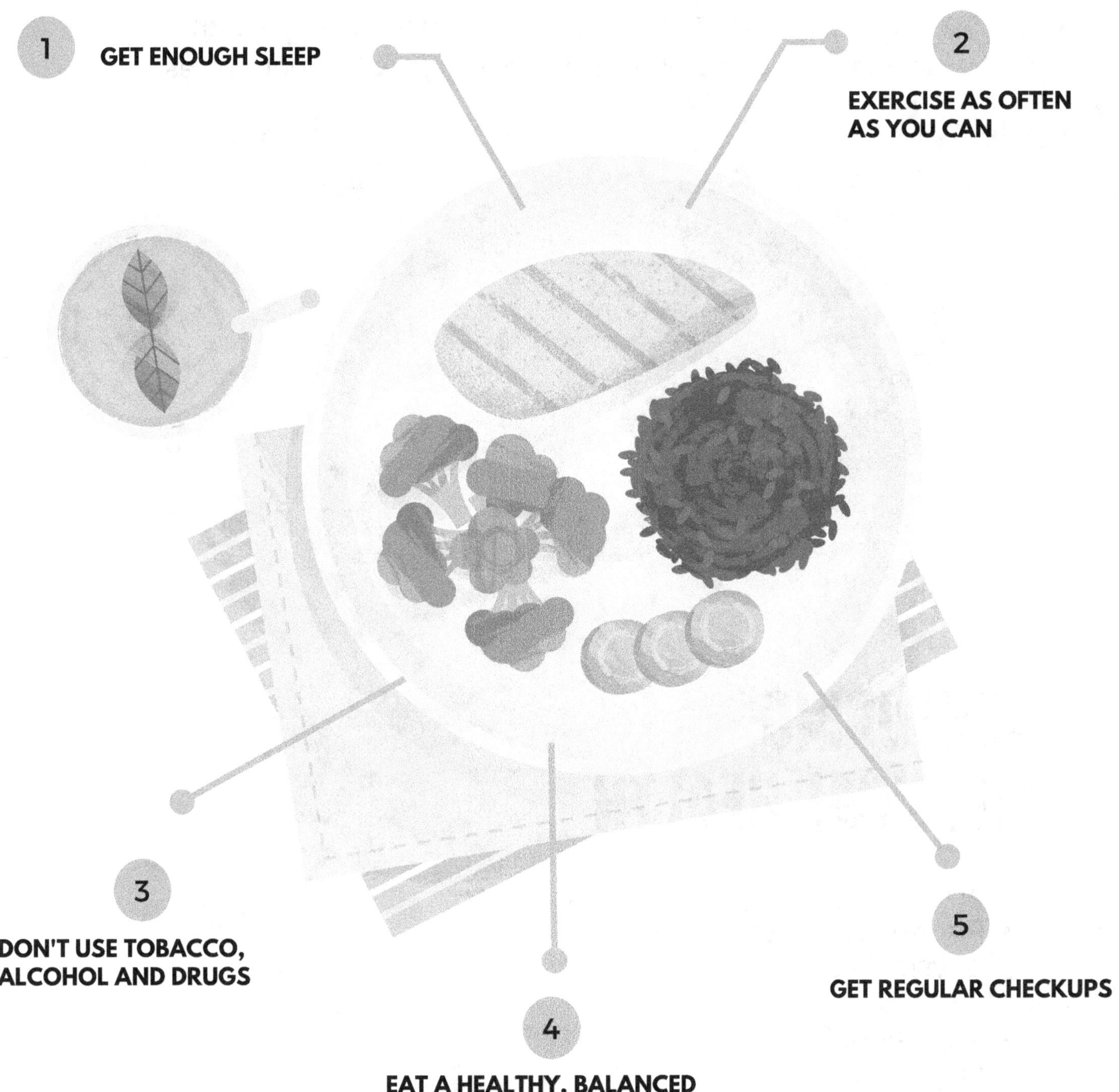

HEALTHY HABITS
for Well-Being

Remember, the journey towards a better life starts with understanding oneself and embracing growth opportunities.

NURTURING PHYSICAL HEALTH

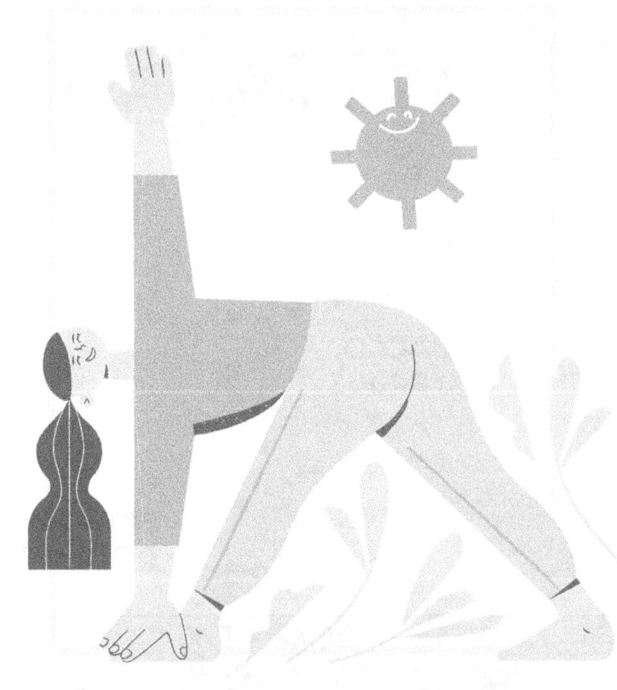

- Prioritize regular exercise and physical activity.

- Maintain a balanced and nutritious diet.

- Get adequate sleep for optimal cognitive and physical functioning.

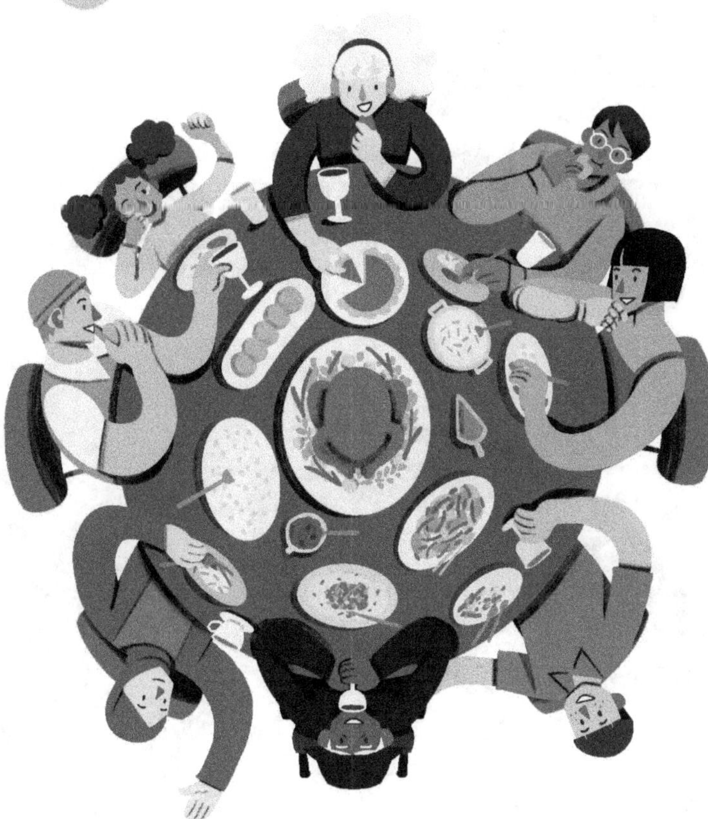

Healthy Eating Tips

for Young Adults

Developing healthy eating habits is a long-term process. Small, gradual changes can lead to significant improvements in your overall health and well-being. Focus on nourishing your body with nutrient-dense foods and making sustainable choices that align with your lifestyle.

01

Incorporating a Variety

Incorporating fruits, vegetables, whole grains, and lean proteins into meals supports overall health and provides essential nutrients for young adults.

02

Limiting Processed Foods,

Sugary beverages and excessive sodium intake can harm maintaining a healthy weight and increase the risk of chronic diseases.

03

Drinking an adequate amount of

Water daily is crucial for hydration, digestion, and maintaining overall well-being.

04

Plan Ahead

Plan your meals and snacks in advance to avoid impulsive and unhealthy food choices. Prepare a grocery list and stock up on nutritious ingredients.

05

Seek Nutritional Guidance

If you have specific dietary needs or concerns, consult with a registered dietitian or nutritionist who can provide personalized advice and guidance.

Healthy Eating Tips

Fruits and Vegetables

Consume a colourful array of fruits and vegetables, as they provide essential vitamins and minerals.

Protein Choices and Healthy Fats

Include lean protein sources like poultry, fish, tofu, and beans in your diet. Limit red and processed meats.

Reduce Sugar and Balanced Meals

Aim for balanced meals that include a variety of food groups: vegetables, fruits, lean proteins, whole grains, and healthy fats.

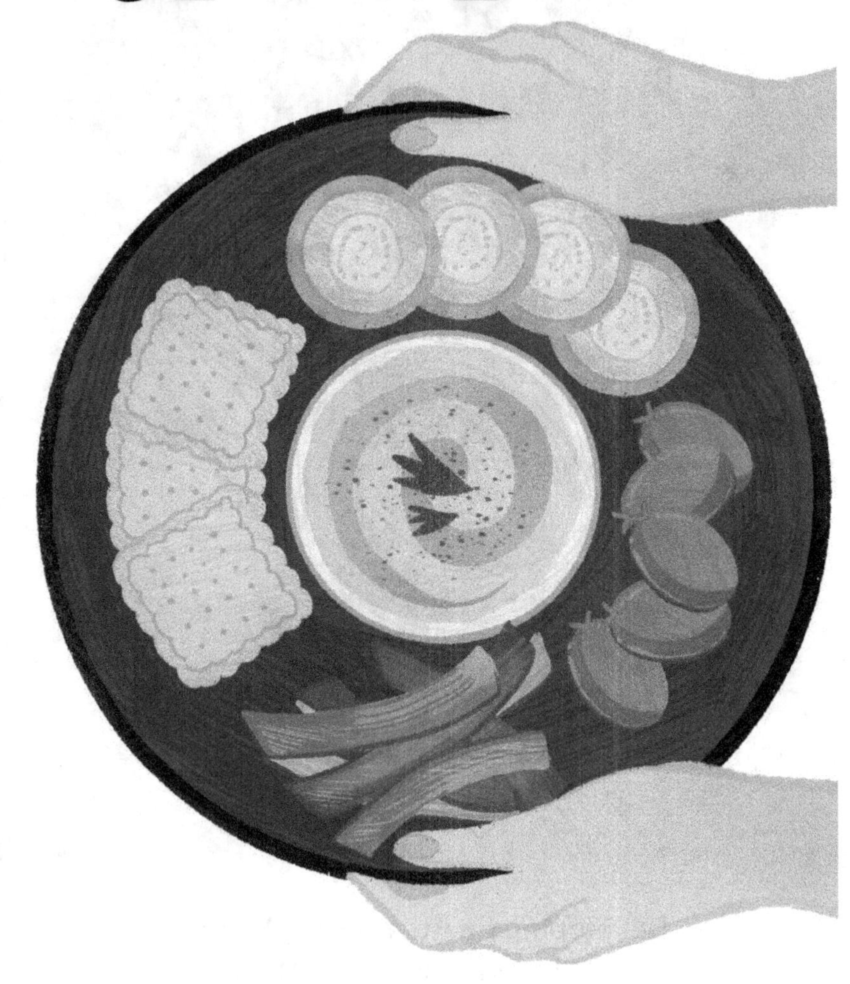

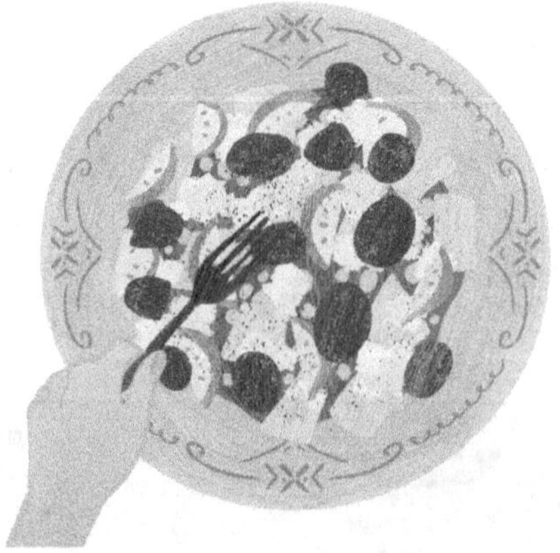

Plan Ahead

Plan your meals and snacks in advance to make healthier choices and avoid impulsive, less nutritious options.

5 Important Nutrients For The Body

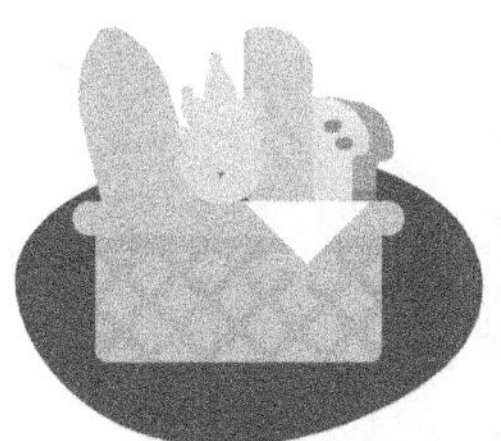

Carbohydrate

This one nutrient has an important role, especially in providing energy to the body. Carbohydrates are needed to provide fuel for the body which converts the glucose component in carbohydrates into energy.

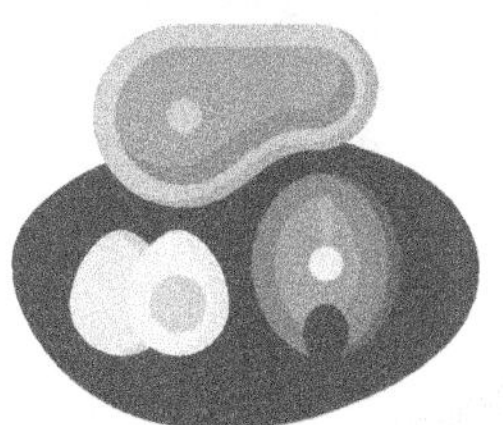

Protein

Protein is a long chain of amino acids which are the basic building blocks of the body. Protein is very good for the health of muscles, bone cells, skin and hair.

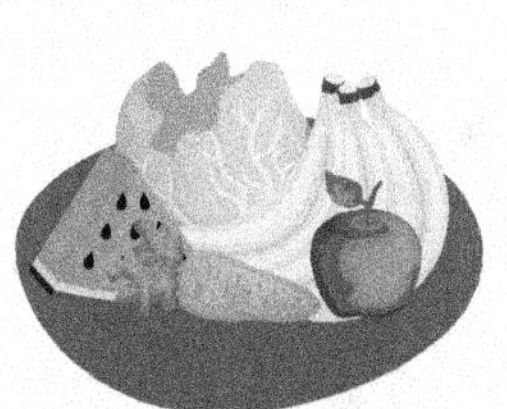

Vitamins

Vitamins are one of the most important nutrients, namely in various chemical processes in the body, maintaining organ function, and increasing the body's immunity against disease.

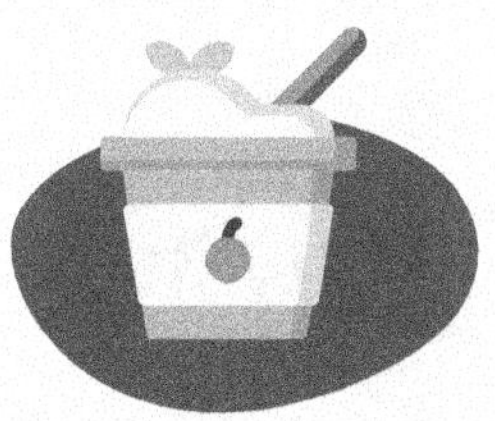

Minerals

Minerals function in building strong bones and teeth, regulate metabolism, and keep the body well hydrated. Some of the minerals that are widely known are calcium, iron, and zinc.

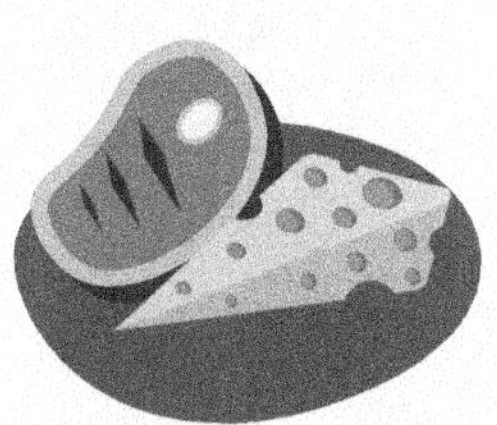

Fats

Fat helps maintain organ function and assists in the process of absorbing nutrients, blood clotting, cell formation, and muscle movement. Even consumption of good fats can help the body control blood sugar, reduce the risk of heart disease, etc.

Healthy Food

FOR YOUR SKIN

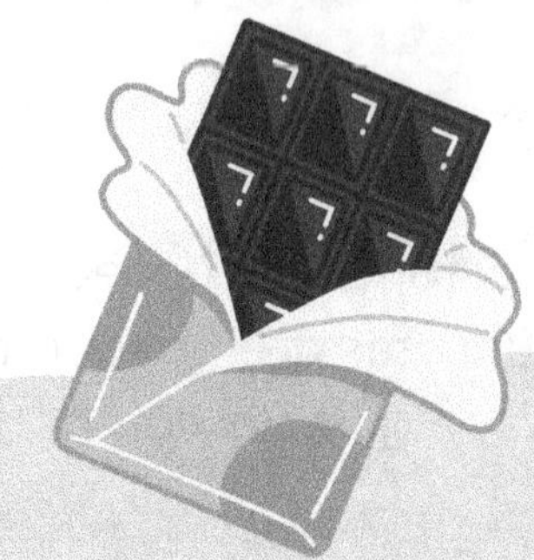

DARK CHOCOLATE

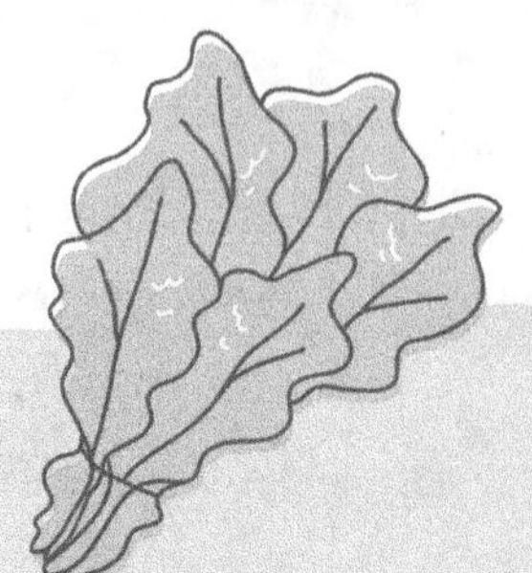

KALE

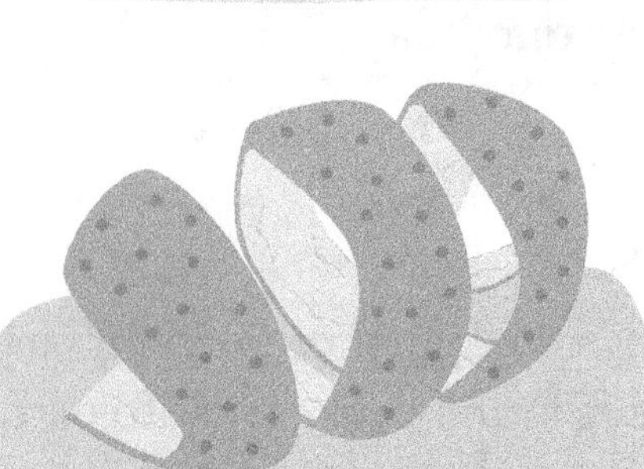

CITRUS PEELS

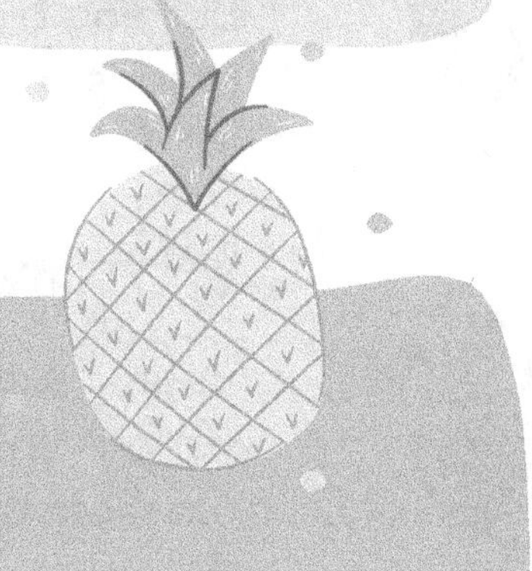

PINEAPPLE

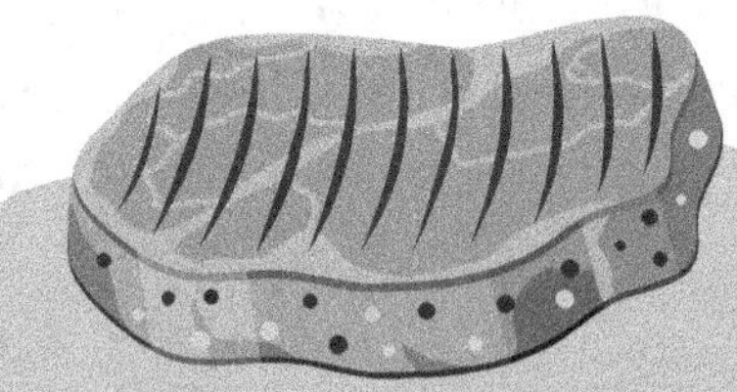

GRASS-FED BEEF

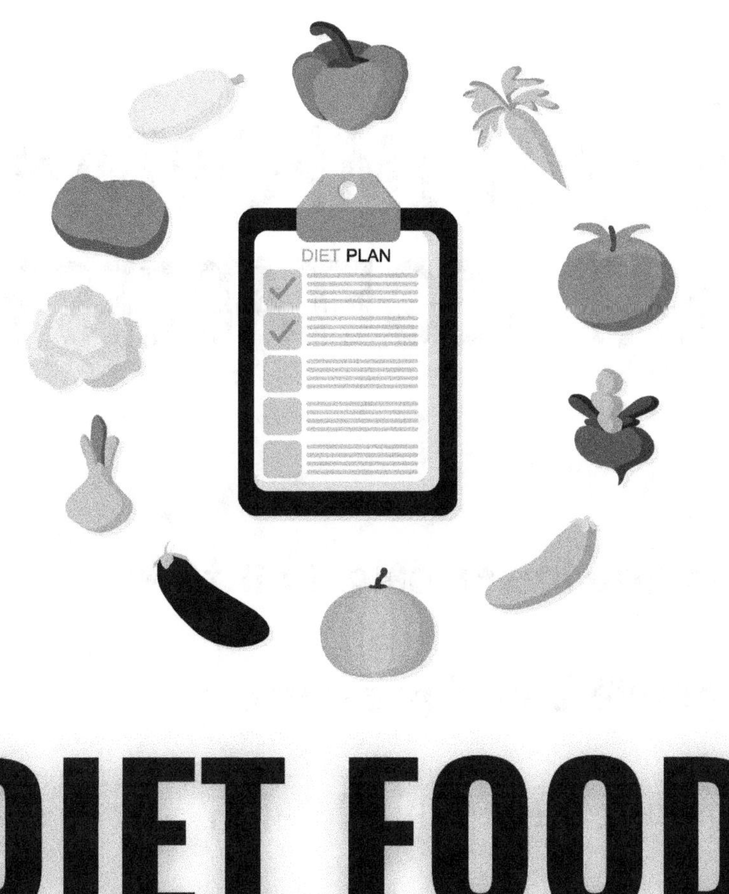

DIET FOOD
Tips

✔ **Eat lots of fruit and veg**

✔ **Do not get thirsty**

✔ **Do not skip breakfast**

WHY IS IT IMPORTANT TO EAT VEGETABLES?

- Help you lower calorie intake
- Improve blood pressure
- Improve digestive health
- Reduce the risk of cancer
- Help keep your immune system strong

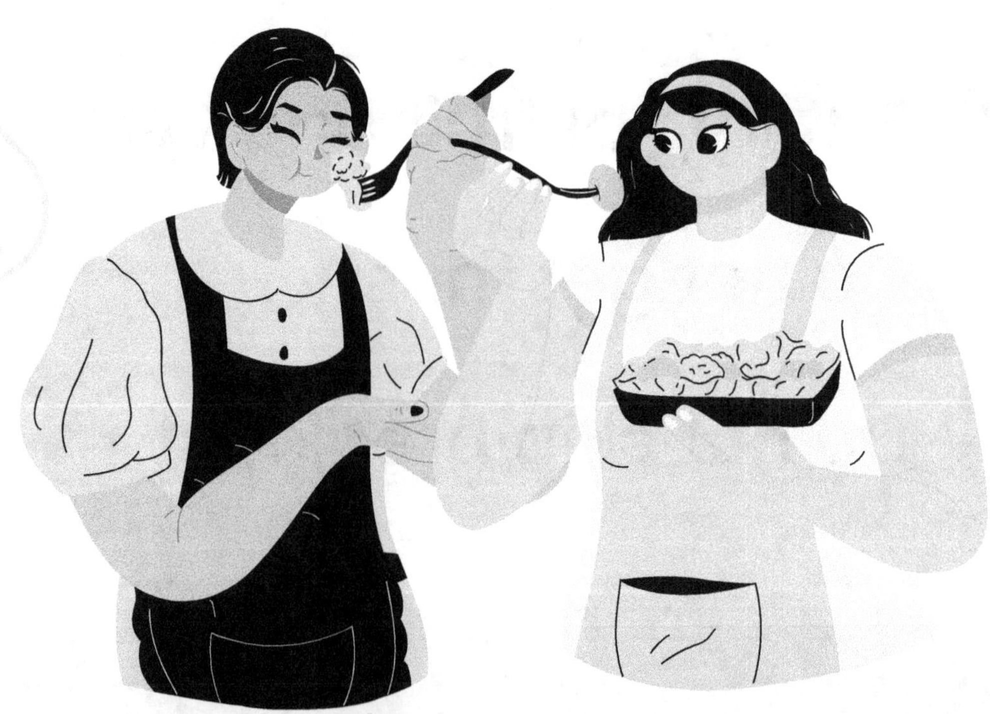

Health Benefits Of
Eating Vegetables
For Your Body

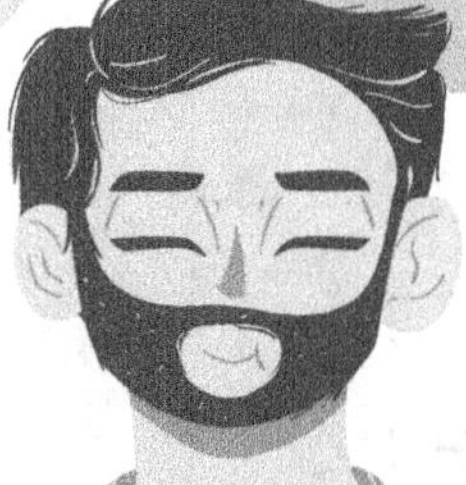

benefits of eating
VEGETABLES

Lorem ipsum dolor sit amet, consectetur adipiscing elit, sed do eiusmod tempor incididunt ut labore et dolore magna aliqua. Ut enim ad minim veniam, quis nostrud exercitation ullamco laboris nisi ut aliquip ex ea commodo consequat.

BENEFITS CONSUMTION VEGETABLES

- Describe Text Here I
- Describe Text Here II
- Describe Text Here III
- Describe Text Here IV

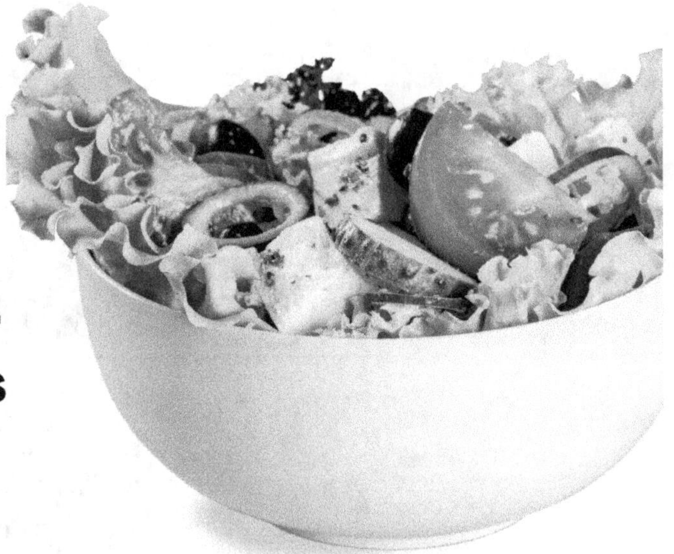

THE NUTRITIONAL CONTENT AVAILABLE IN VEGETABLES

- Describe Text Here I
- Describe Text Here II
- Describe Text Here III
- Describe Text Here IV

THE BENEFITS OF FRUIT

PINEAPPLE

Rich in potassium, calcium, vitamin C, beta carotene, thiamin, B6, as well as soluble and insoluble fiber.

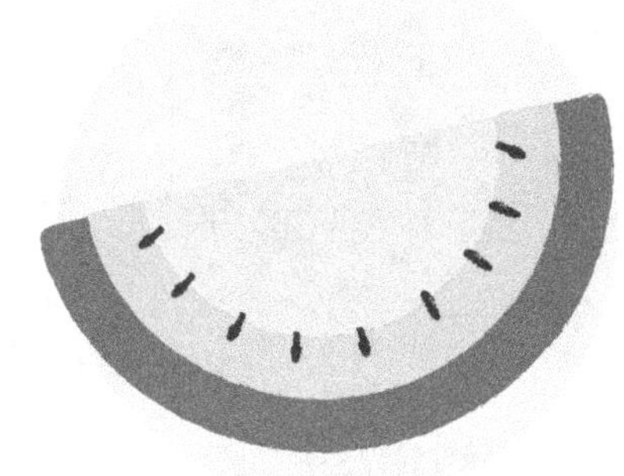

WATERMELON

Helps prevent kidney disorders, high blood pressure, the prevention of cancer, diabetes

ORANGE

Boosts immune system function, reduce signs of aging, protect against cancer, and boost cellular repair.

LEMON

Has nourishing elements like vitamin C, vitamin B6, vitamin A, vitamin E, folate, niacin thiamin, and riboflavin.

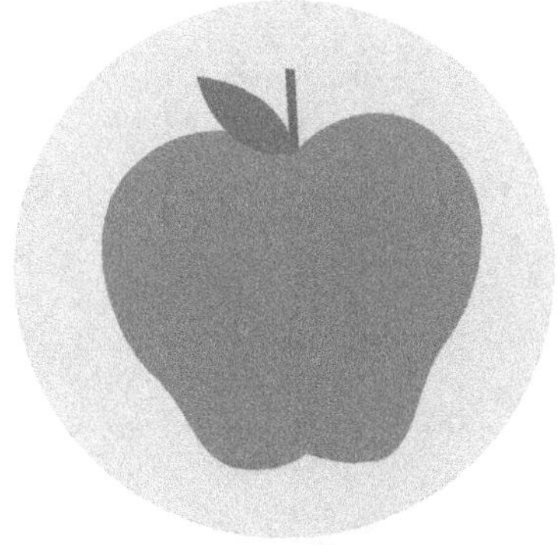

APPLE

Helps improve digestion, prevention of stomach disorders, gallstones, constipation, liver disorders.

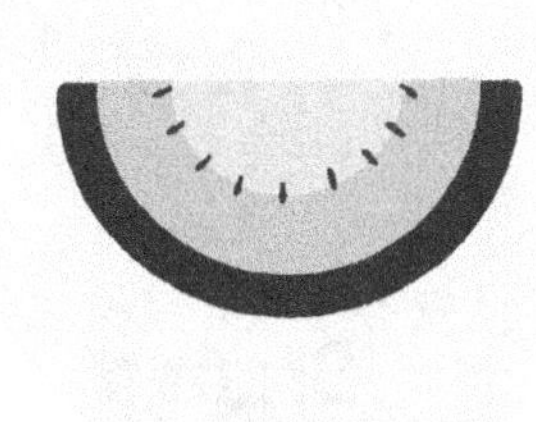

KIWI

An excellent source of vitamin C, vitamin A, folate, vitamin E, and vitamin K. Has antioxidant properties.

BENEFITS OF FRUIT
and its contents

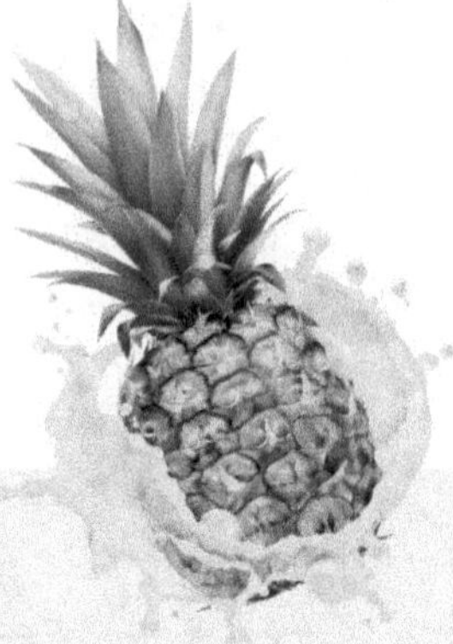

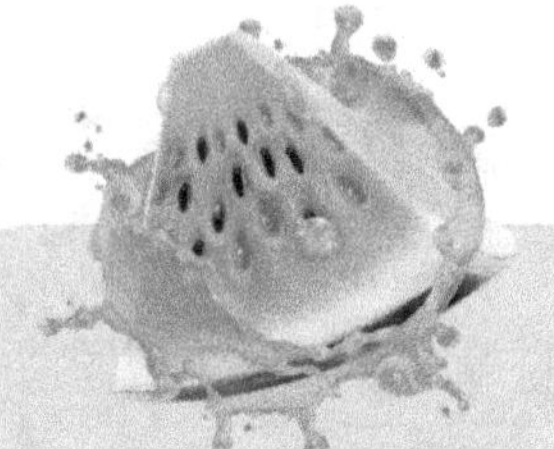

Water Melon

Watermelon contains vitamin A & C and the antioxidant lycopene. Watermelon can prevent dehydration and good for heart health.

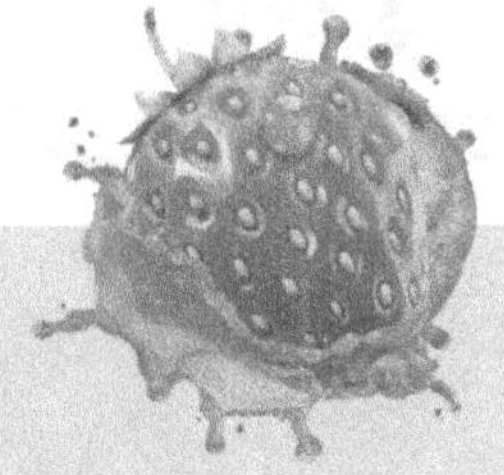

Pinneaple

Pineapple is rich in antioxidants and contains vitamin C which is good for increasing endurance and preventing various diseases.

Strawberry

Strawberries contain vitamin C and are rich in antioxidants, which are helpful in reducing the growth of cancerous cells.

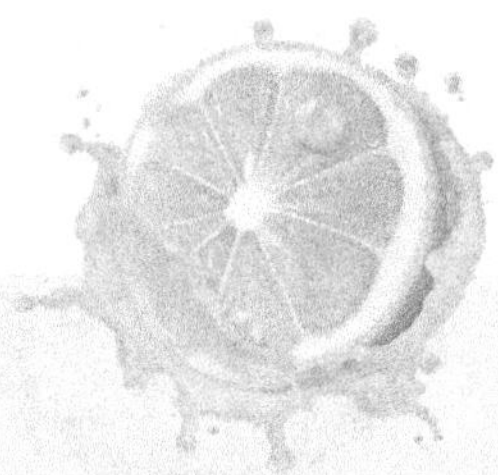

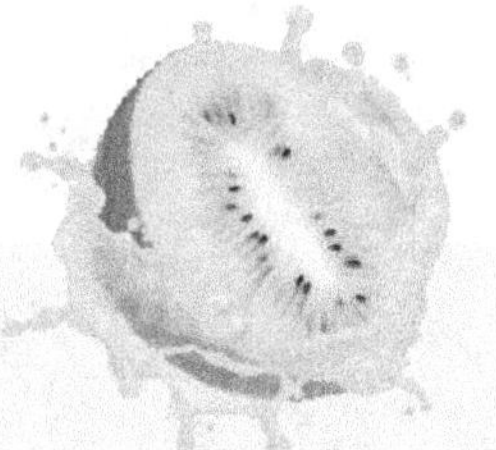

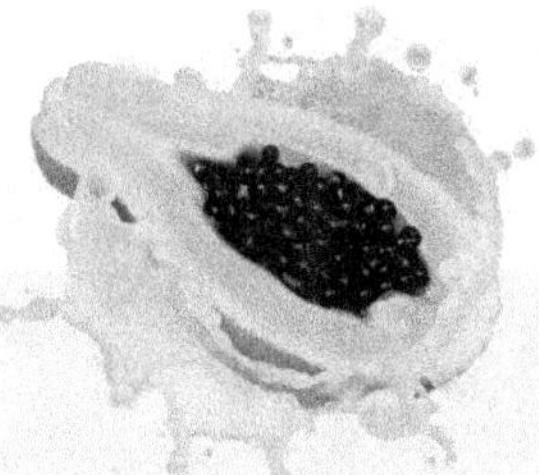

Orange

Oranges are a source of vitamin C, contain vitamin B1, folate, and potassium which are useful for boosting the body's immunity.

Kiwi

The content of vitamin C in kiwi fruit is beneficial for skin health, can prevent premature aging and overcome acne.

Papaya

Papaya contains two proteolytic enzymes, papain and chymopapain, which is helpful for protein digestion and helps digestive problems.

LOOK GREAT & FEEL HEALTHY

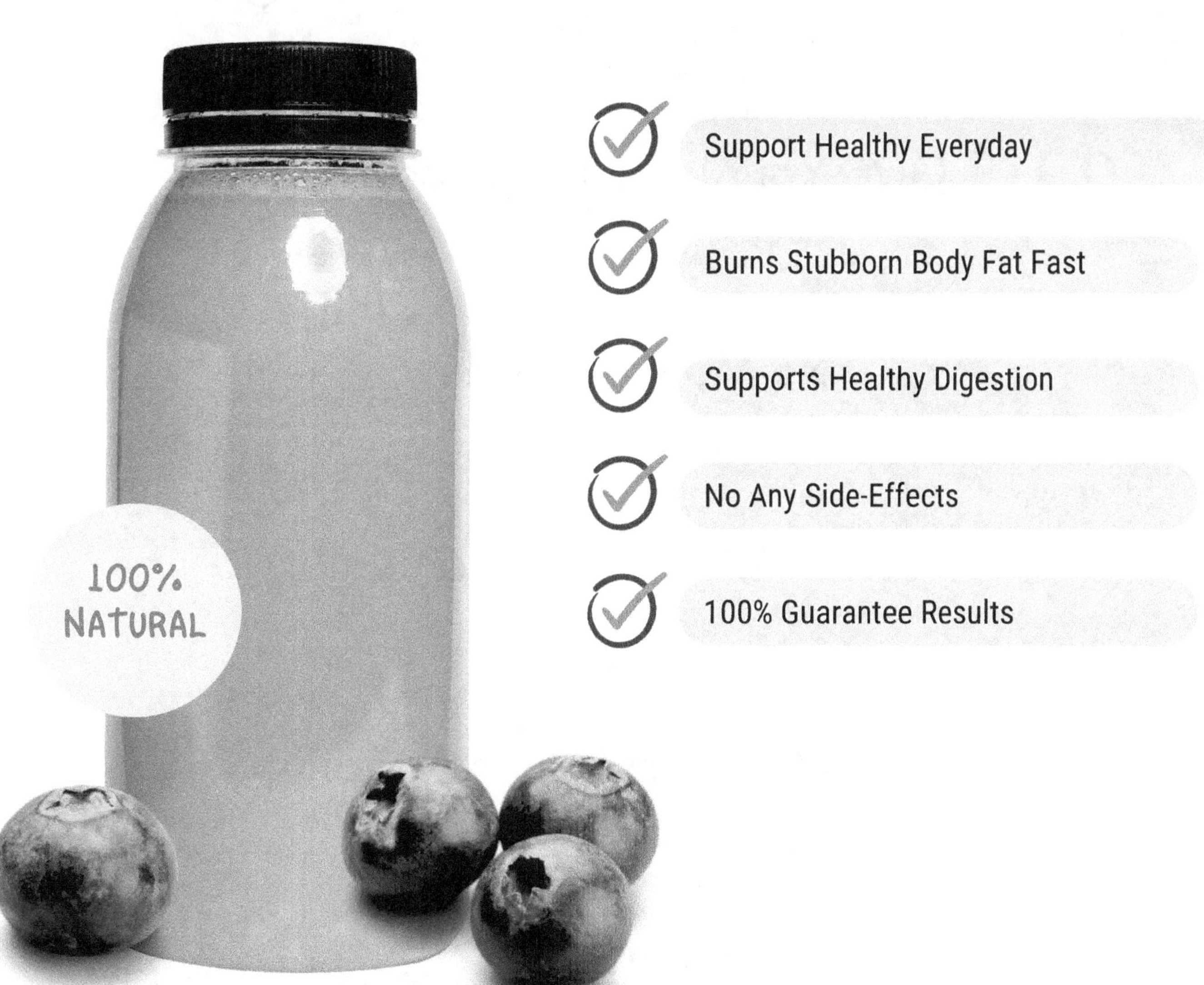

- Support Healthy Everyday
- Burns Stubborn Body Fat Fast
- Supports Healthy Digestion
- No Any Side-Effects
- 100% Guarantee Results

Surprice Benefit Of
Strawberry

Give Your Immunity A Boots

No More Wrinkles

Aid In Weight Management

Maintain Your Healthy Vision

Benefits of Strawberries for Health

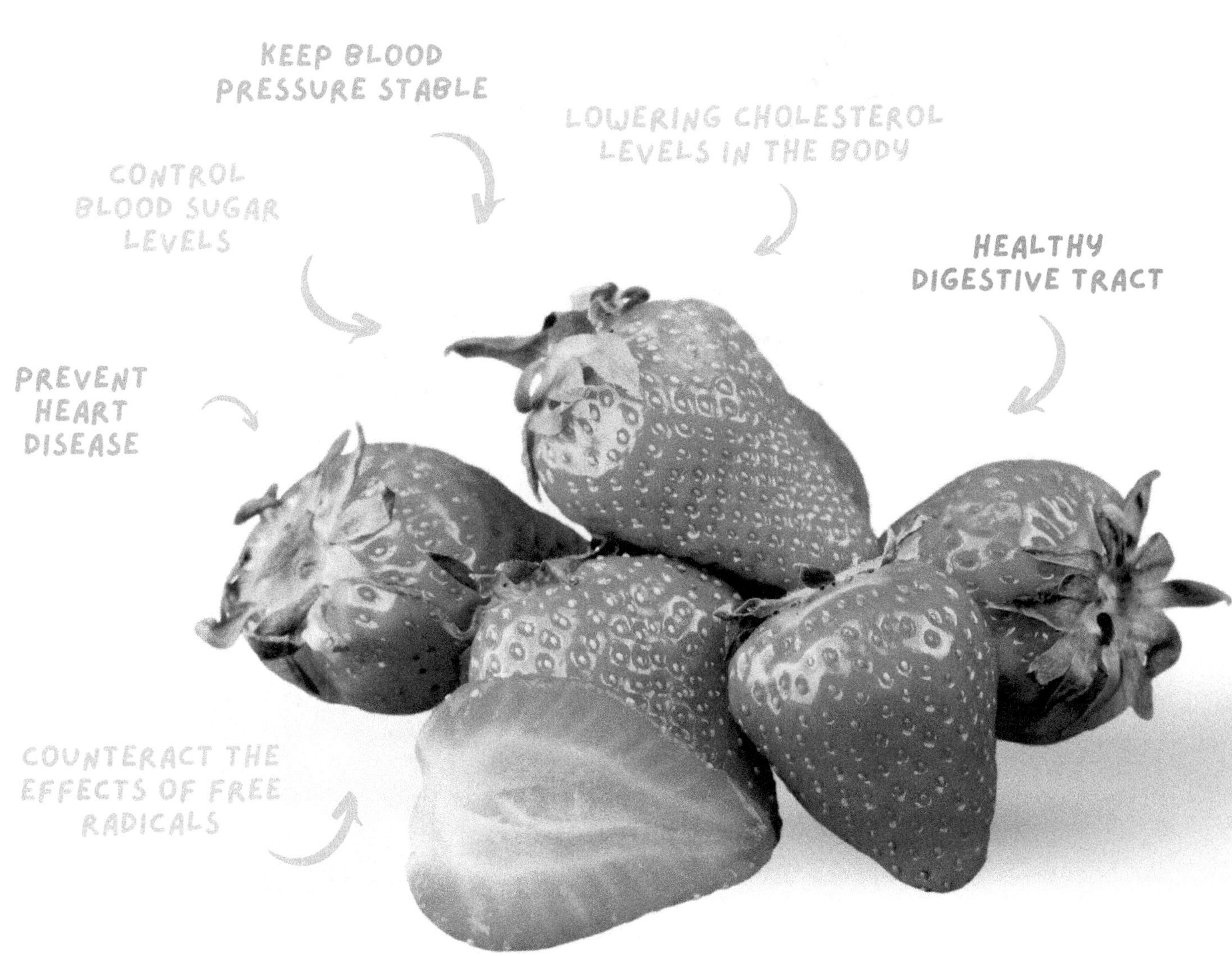

BENEFITS OF BANANAS FOR BODY HEALTH

- AS A SOURCE OF ENERGY

- MAINTAIN A HEALTHY HEART AND BLOOD VESSELS

- PREVENTS CELL AND TISSUE DAMAGE

- REDUCE THE RISK OF KIDNEY DISEASE

- REDUCING NAUSEA DURING PREGNANCY

- MAINTAIN DIGESTIVE TRACT HEALTH

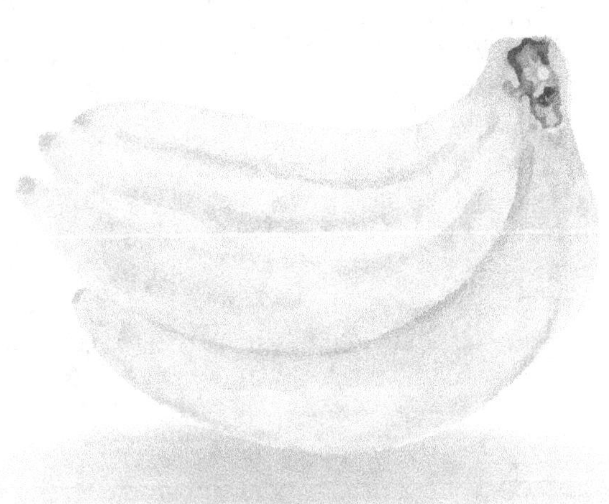

BENEFITS OF PEARS FOR HEALTH

- Improve skin health

- Helps maintain weight

- Improve digestive health

- Helps maintain healthy nerves

- Lowers the risk of developing type 2 diabetes

- Increase endurance

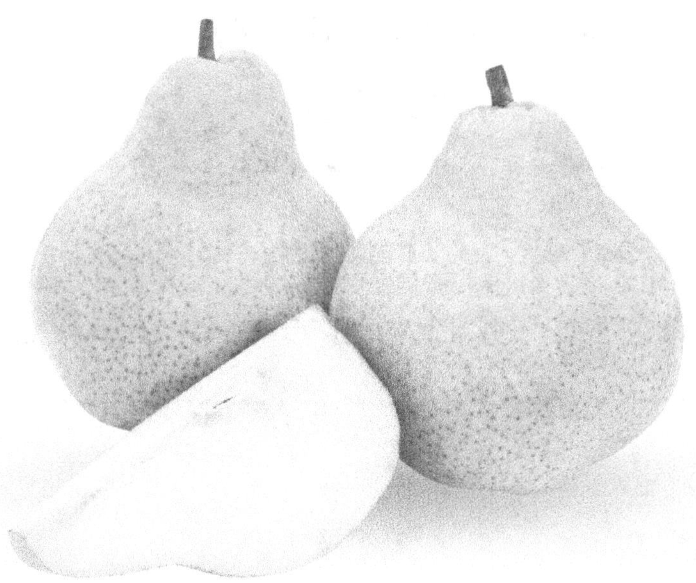

THE BENEFITS OF AVOCADO

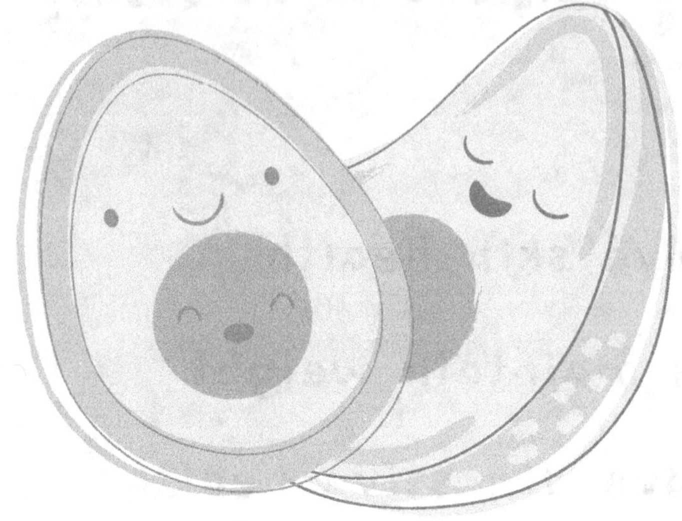

Versatile and delicious ingredient

Excellent source of nutrients

Beneficial for gut health

A smart choice during pregnancy and breastfeeding

BENEFITS OF GRAPES FOR HEALTH

- Reduce the risk of diabetes

- Prevent cancer

- Improve memory

- Reduce the risk of diabetes

- Lowering high blood pressure

- Overcoming blood vessel and heart disorders
- Reducing the symptoms of chronic venous insufficiency

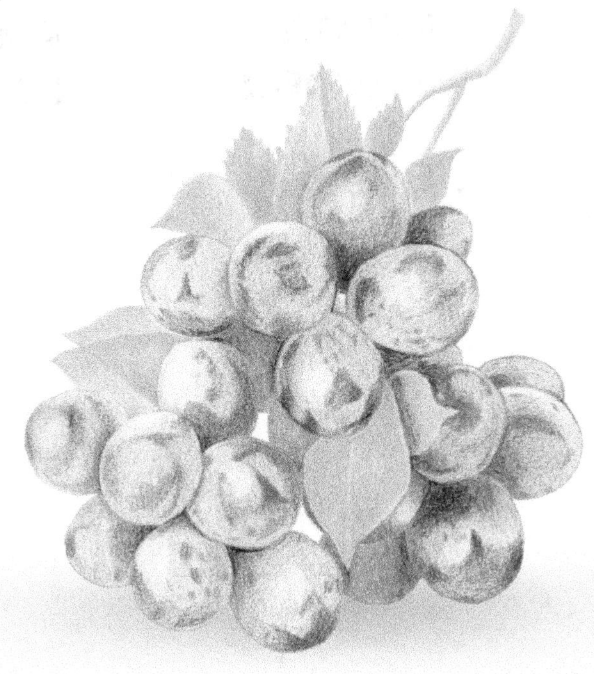

BENEFITS OF PINEAPPLE FOR HEALTH

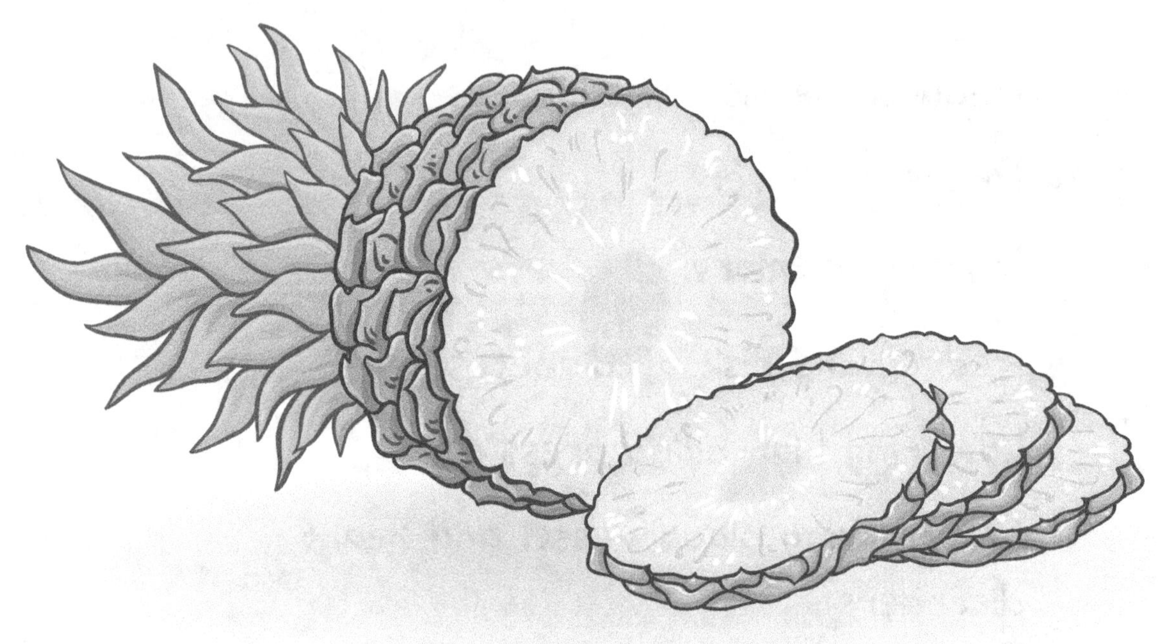

- BOOST IMMUNITY
- IMPROVE CARDIOVASCULAR HEALTH
- OVERCOME DIGESTIVE DISORDERS
- REDUCE INFLAMMATION
- HELPS MAINTAIN HEALTHY SKIN AND BONES
- LOSE WEIGHT

HEALTH BENEFITS OF
Lychee Fruit

maintain healthy skin

improve the digestive system

provide vitamin c content

provide iron content

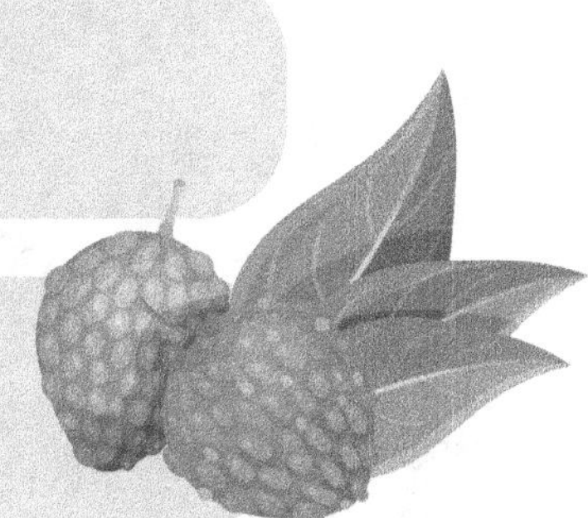

good for the health of pregnant women

maintain blood sugar levels in the body

prevent us from chronic disease

help lose weight

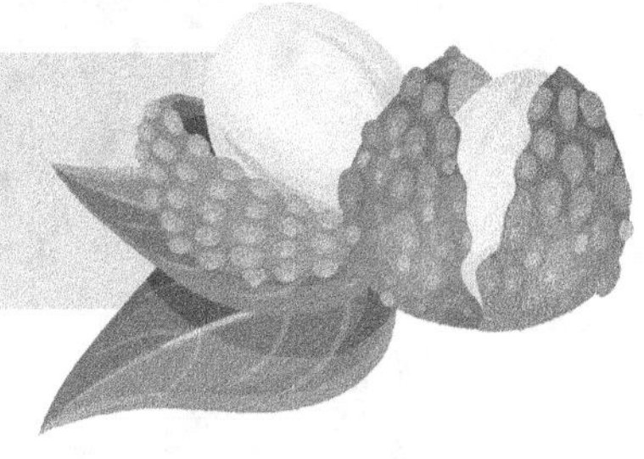

Benefits of
CACTUS

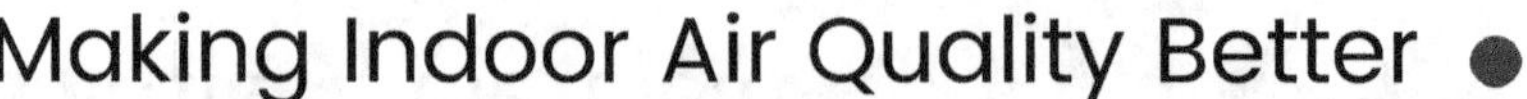

- Making Indoor Air Quality Better
- Can improve mood
- As home decoration
- Minimum maintenance
- Help to focus

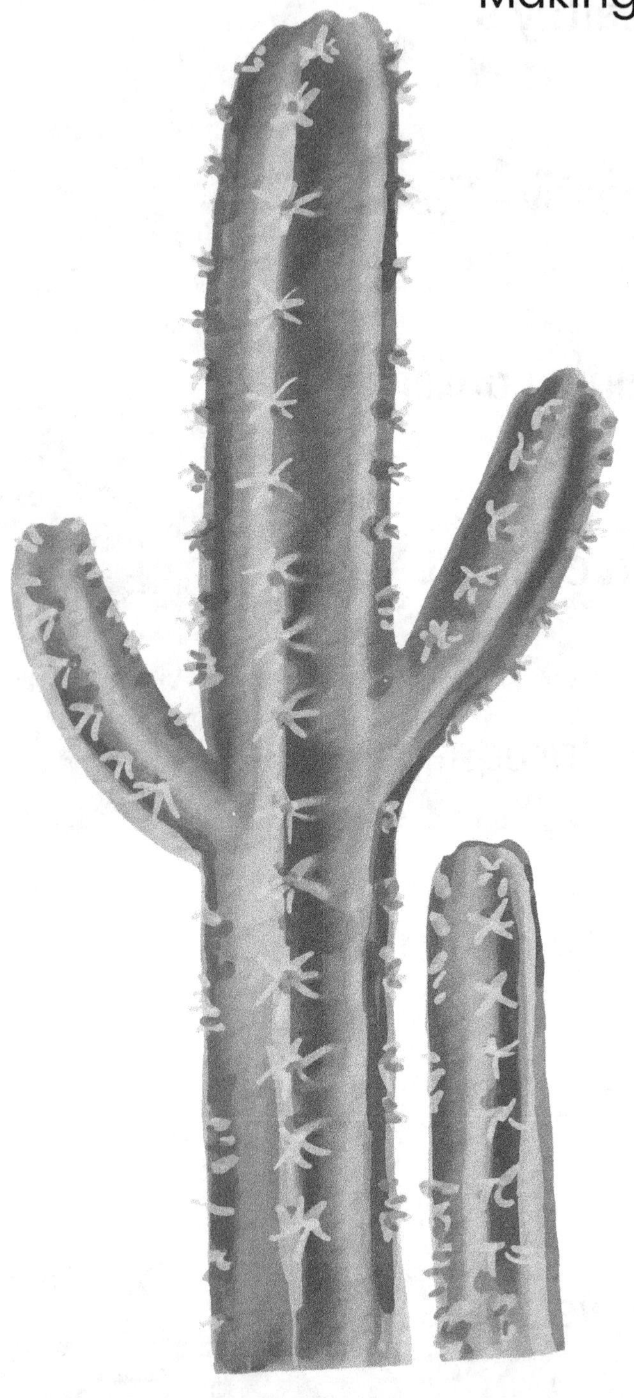

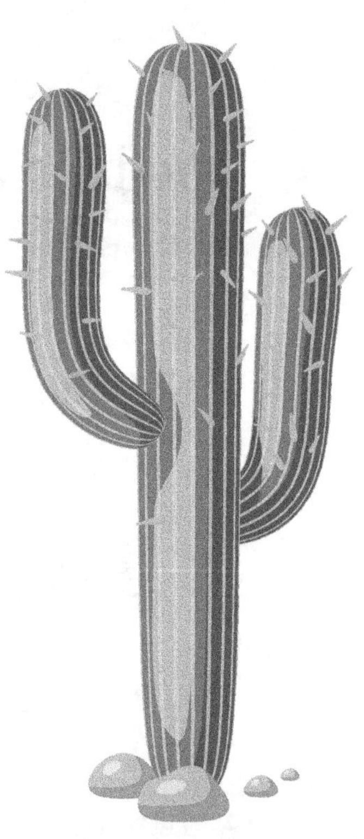

BENEFITS OF RED DRAGON FRUIT

Prevent anemia

Prevent migraines

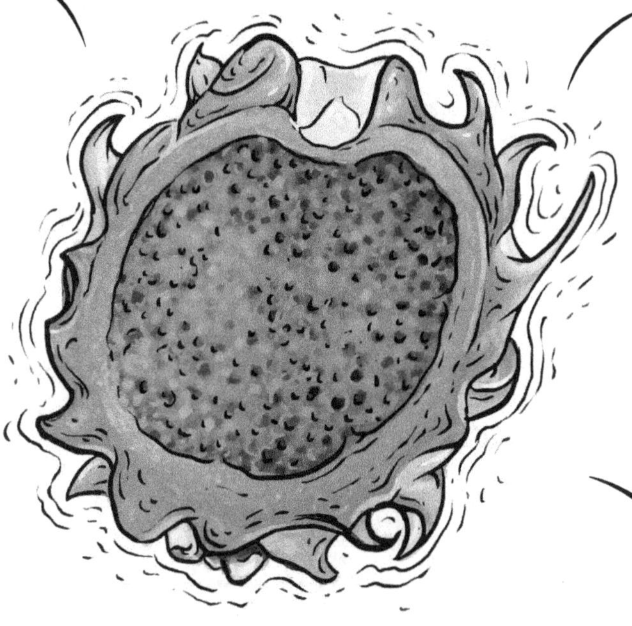

Maintain bone health

Protects the body from free radicals

Stimulate the formation of collagen

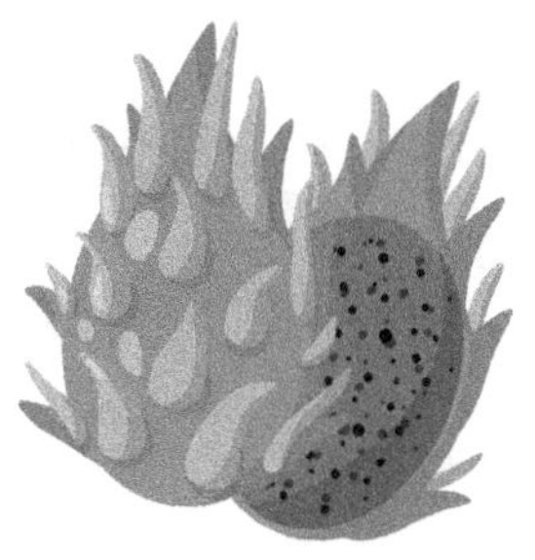

THE BENEFITS OF AVOCADO

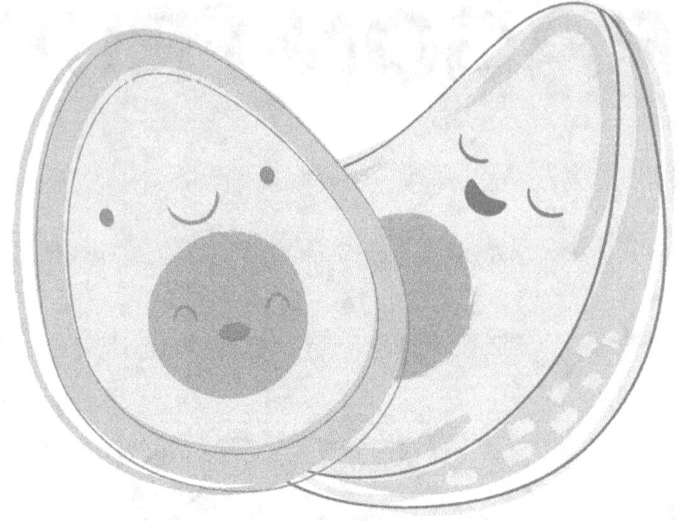

Versatile and delicious ingredient

Excellent source of nutrients

Beneficial for gut health

A smart choice during pregnancy and breastfeeding

BENEFITS OF JUICING IN THE MORNING

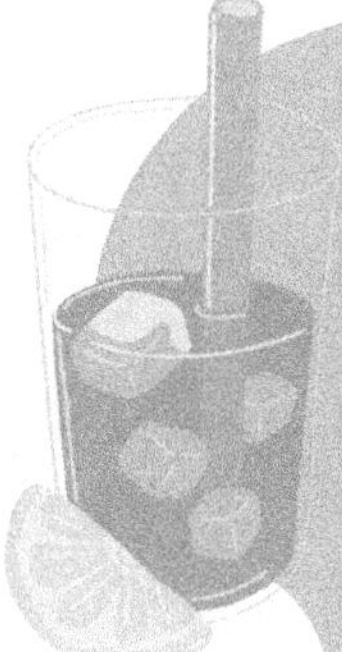

Improve Digestion
The fruit is rich in fiber, which is good for digestion and minimizes constipation.

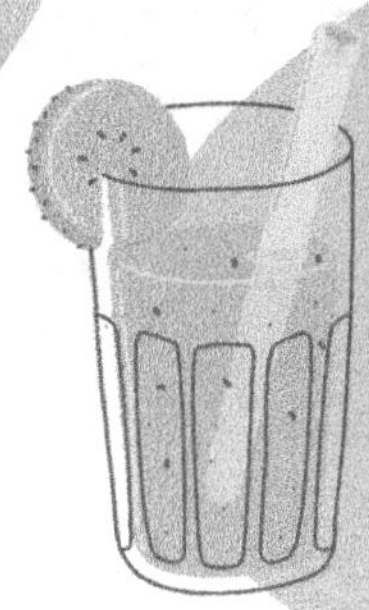

Prevent Cancer
Fruit contains antioxidants that can fight cancer cells.

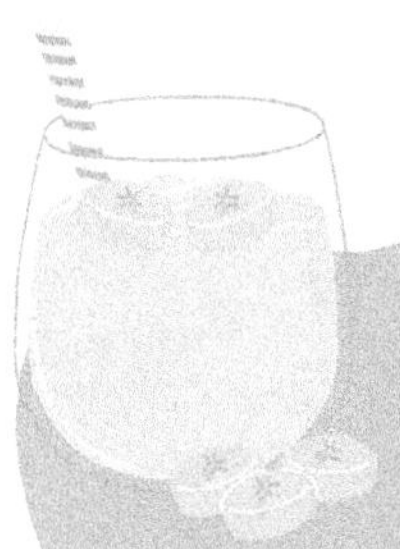

Help Lose Weight
Nutrition and fiber in fruit is good for maintaining ideal body weight.

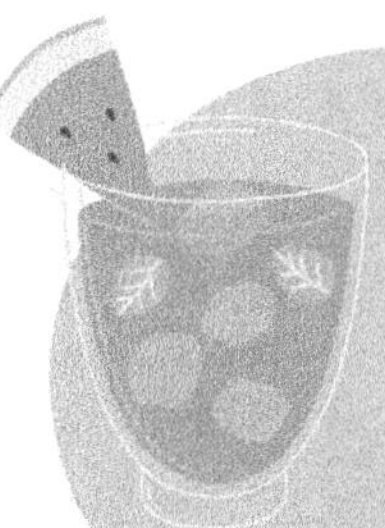

Medicine To Stay Young
The fruit contains vitamin C that is good for skin growth, regenerates dead skin cells.

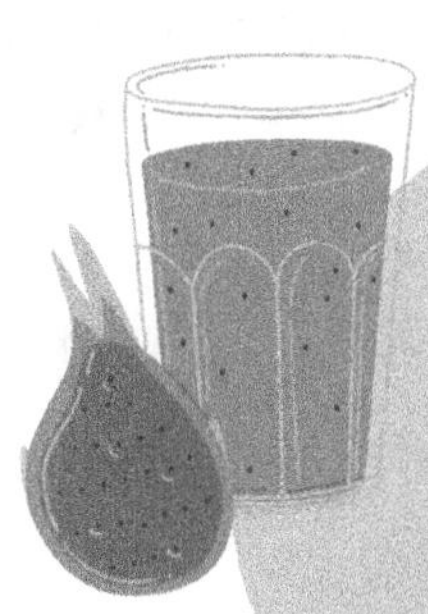

Energy Sources
Fruit contains various kinds of vitamins, fiber and minerals that can help the body's energy formation process.

benefits of garlic

FOR NUTRITION AND HEALTH

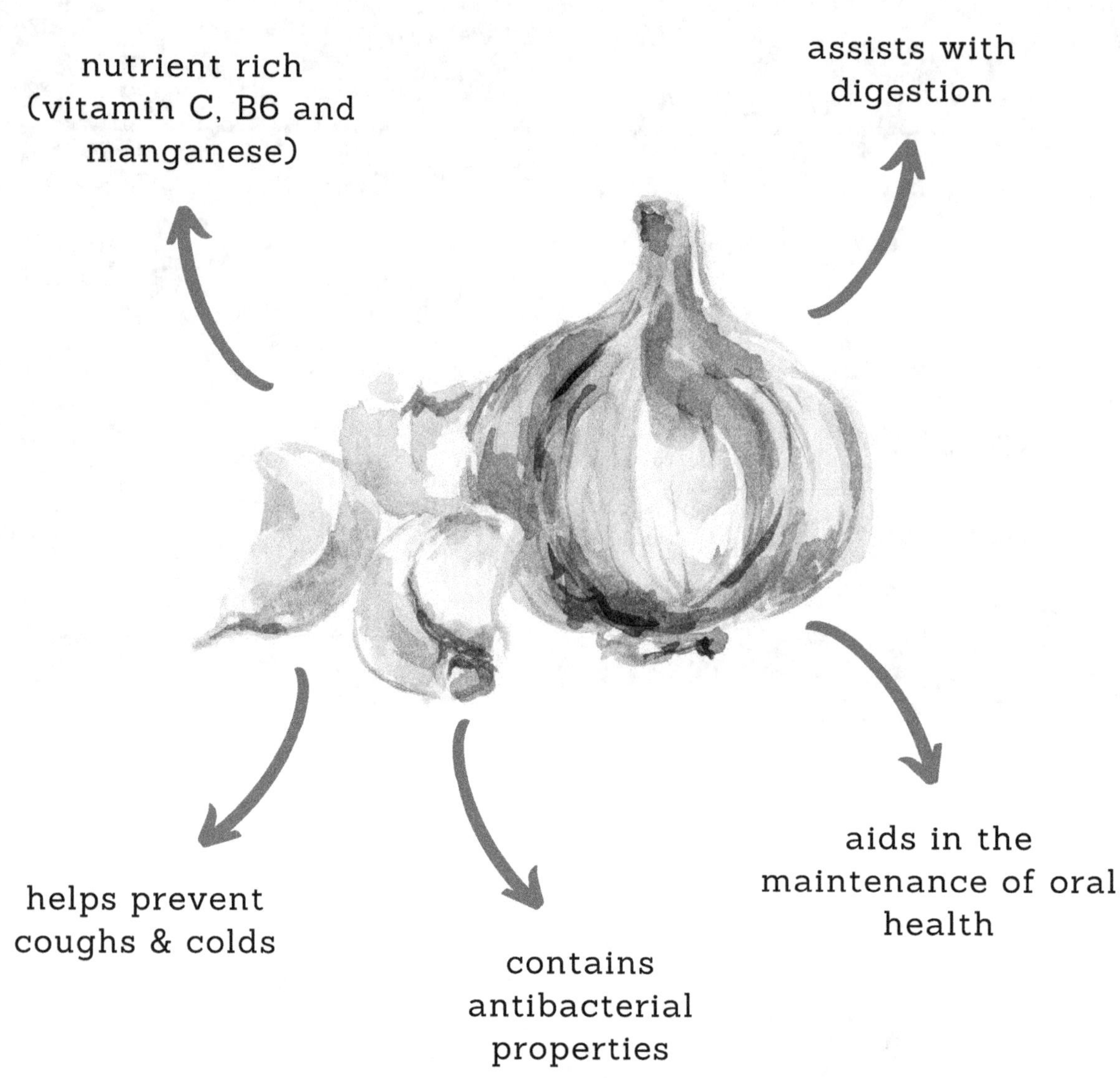

4 BENEFITS OF TOMATOES FOR THE BODY

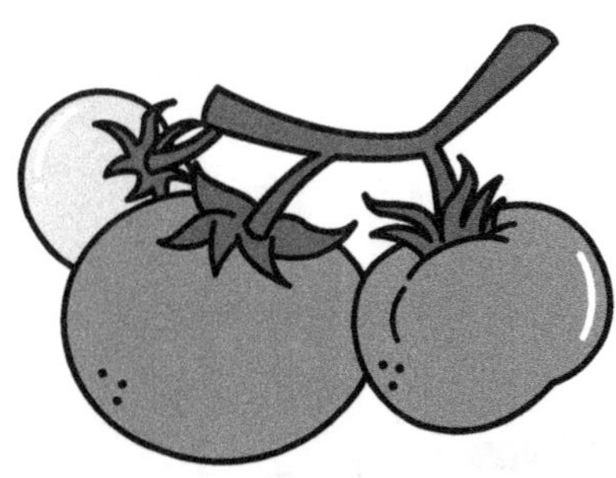

01 RICH IN ANTIOXIDANTS

Tomatoes are packed with antioxidants like lycopene, which can help reduce the risk of chronic diseases and protect cells from damage caused by free radicals.

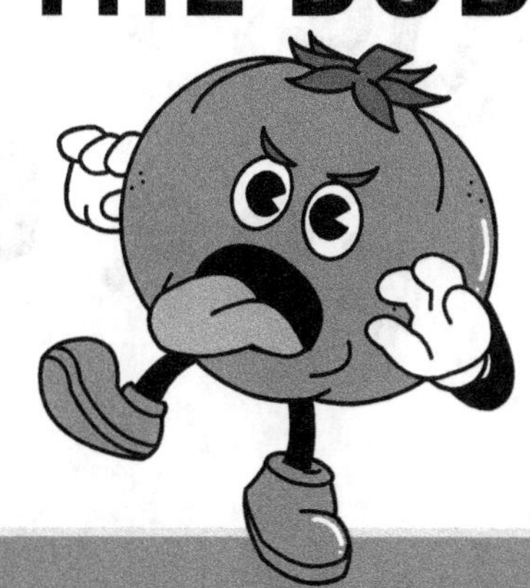

02 SUPPORTS HEART HEALTH

The nutrients in tomatoes, including potassium and vitamin C, contribute to heart health by helping to lower blood pressure and reduce the risk of heart disease.

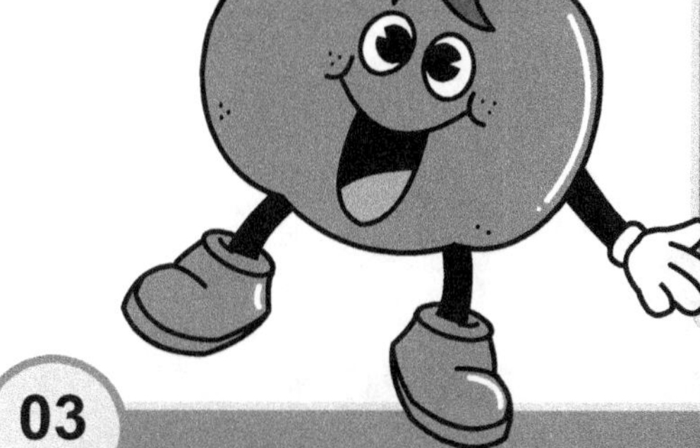

03 IMPROVES SKIN HEALTH

The high content of vitamins A and C in tomatoes can promote healthier skin by supporting collagen production, which aids in maintaining skin elasticity and reducing signs of aging.

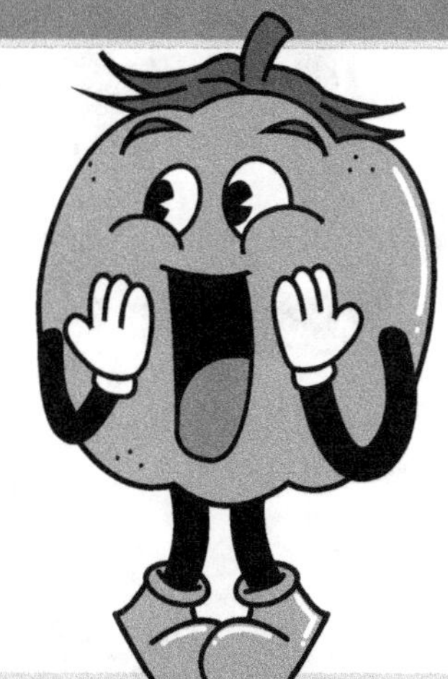

04 AIDS DIGESTION

Tomatoes are a good source of fiber, which supports healthy digestion and can prevent constipation. They also contain compounds that may help prevent digestive issues.

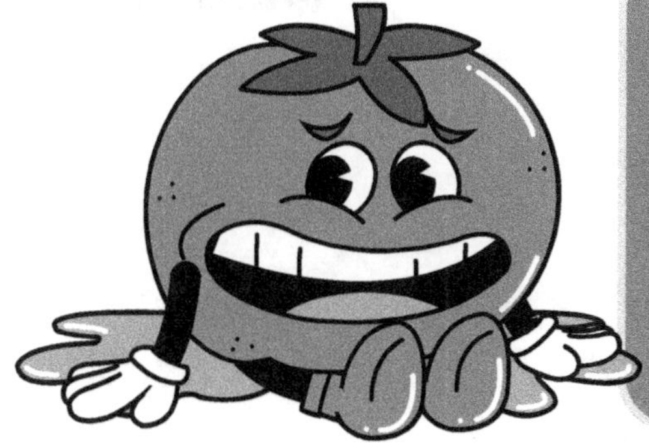

CUCUMBER BENEFITS FOR BODY HEALTH

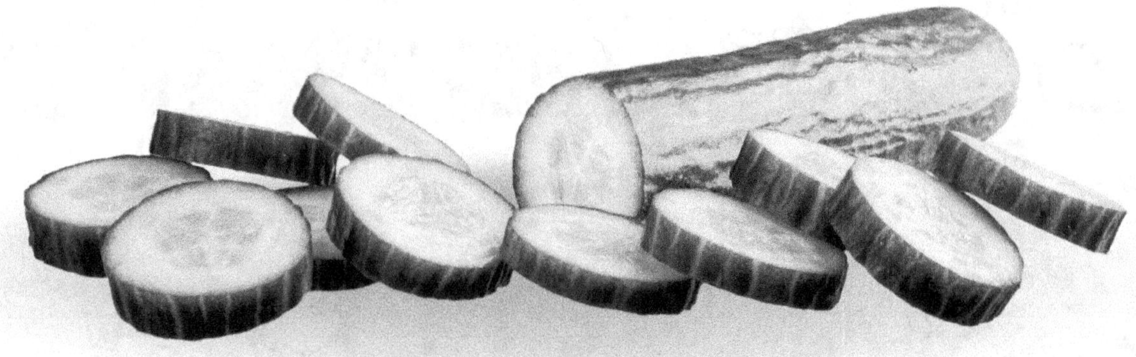

BENEFITS OF

Green Tea

Improves Mood

Contains Healthy Bioactive Compounds

Lower Cholesterol

Reducing Inflammation

Help You Lose Weight

Can Help With Stress & Anxiety

Health Benefits Of
HONEY

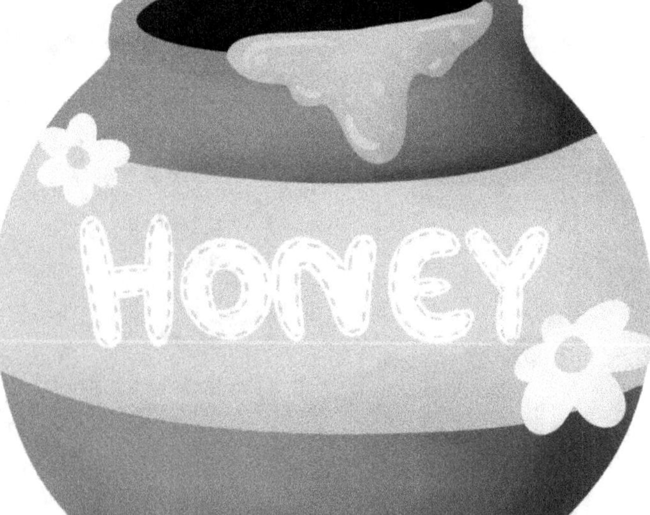

Best Vegetable in Winter

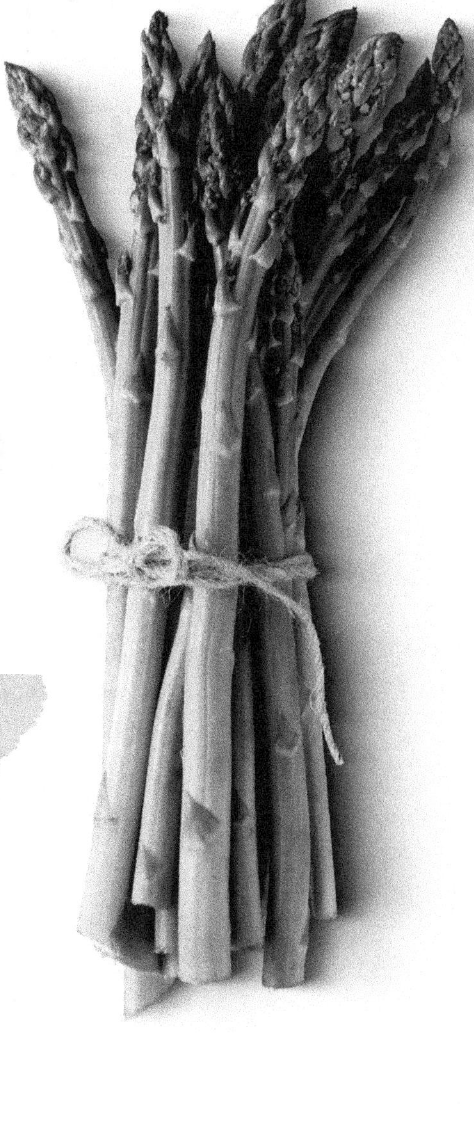

Asparagus

1. **Many nutrients but few calories**

2. **Good source of antioxidants**

3. **Can improve digestive health**

4. **Easy to add to your diet**

5. **Helps lower blood pressure**

Nutrition

Calories:	27 kcal
Protein:	3 g
Total fat:	0.16 g
Fiber:	3 g
Potassium:	273 mg
Folate:	70.2 mcg

(One cup (135 g) of uncooked asparagus)

Veg vs Non-Veg

A never ending debate

VEGETARIANISM AND NON-VEGETARIANISM ARE TWO CONTRASTING DIETARY LIFESTYLES WITH DIFFERING OPINIONS.

Today we will know which one is actually more beneficial for us.

Let's find out who is
a vegetarian

Now let's know who is
non-vegetarian.

VEG	NON VEG
HEALTH	**HEALTH**
A plant-based diet is healthier.	Meat is a good source of protein and essential nutrients.
ANIMAL WELFARE	**NUTRITIONAL VALUE**
A vegetarian diet promotes the welfare of animals.	Meat is a rich source of nutrients such as iron, zinc, and vitamin B12.
ANIMAL WELFARE	**NUTRITIONAL VALUE**
Taste: Plant-based foods can be just as delicious with the proper preparation.	Taste: Meat is absolutely delicious.
AFFORDABILITY	**PERSONAL CHOICE**
Plant-based foods can be more affordable and accessible than meat.	Individuals have the right to choose what they want to eat based.

HEALTH
Tips

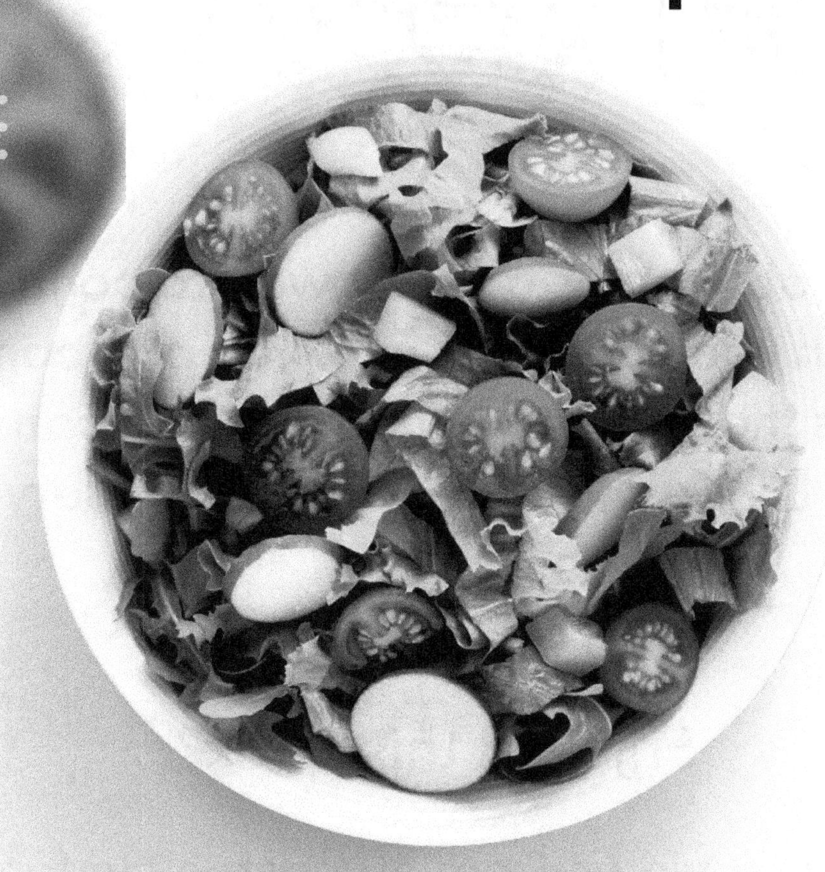

- ✅ Eat healthy!

- ✅ Do a light exercise for 15 min everyday

- ✅ Get enough sleep

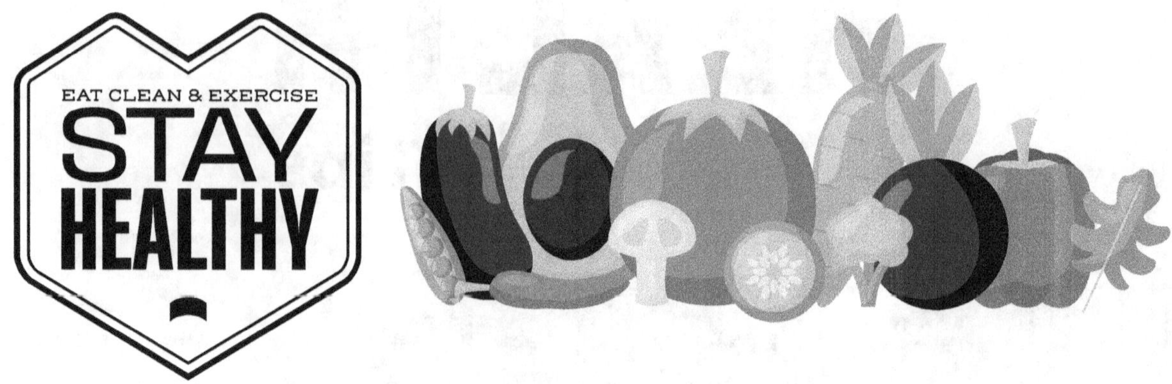

Cooking at home is a great way to control your diet: When you cook at home, you can control the ingredients that go into your food. This can help you to avoid unhealthy additives and preservatives.

Enjoyed this book?

Positive reviews from awesome customers like you help others to feel confident about choosing Maples Book Solutions too.

Could you take 60 seconds to go to Amazon platform and share your happy experiences?

We will be forever grateful. Thank you in advance for helping us out!